GESTATIONAL DIABETES TESTING: YOUR ANSWERS TO THE WHAT? WHEN? AND HOW?

I0116175

BY MATHEA FORD, RDN, LD

BABY STEPS FOR GESTATIONAL DIABETES, VOLUME 3

PURPOSE AND INTRODUCTION

What I have found through the emails and requests of my readers is that it is difficult to find information about a gestational diabetes program that is actionable. I want you to know that is what I intend to provide in all my books. You can take this information from the book and with immediate action you will have a better outcome in your life.

I wrote this module with you in mind: the mom to be with gestational diabetes who does not know where to start or can't seem to get the answers that you need from other sources. This book will provide information that is applicable to a gestational diabetes mom.

Who am I? I am a registered dietitian in the USA who has been working with kidney patients for my entire 15 + years of experience. I was also in your shoes, as a mom to be with gestational diabetes (and now 2 children who are 7 &9) Find all my books on Amazon on my author page: http://www.amazon.com/Mathea-Ford/e/B008E1E7IS/

My goals are simple – to give some answers and to create an understanding of what is typical. In this series for Baby Steps For Gestational Diabetes, I will take you through the different parts of being a woman with gestational diabetes. It will not necessarily be what happens in your case, as everyone is an individual. I may simplify things in an effort to write them so that I feel you can learn the most from the information. This may mean that I don't say the exact things that your doctor would say. If you don't understand, please ask your doctor.

I want you to know, I am not a medical doctor and I am not aware of your particular condition. Information in this book is current as of publication, but may or may not have changed.

This book is not meant to substitute for medical treatment for you, your friends, your caregivers, or your family members. You should not base treatment decisions solely on what is contained in this module. Develop your treatment plan with your doctors, nurses and the other medical professionals on your team. I recommend that you double-check any information with your medical team to verify if it applies to you.

In other words, I am not responsible for your medical care. I am providing this module for information and entertainment purposes, not medical diagnoses. Please consult with your doctor about any questions that you have about your particular case.

© 2013 Healthy Diet Menus For You, LLC, www.gestationaldiabetesdietmealplan.com , All Rights Reserved. No reproduction without author's written permission

We do understand that babies are both male and female, but in the interest of making sure that you can clearly distinguish mom we refer to the baby as he.

TABLE OF CONTENTS

DETECTION AND MANAGEMENT OF GESTATIONAL DIABETES

Gestational diabetes mellitus (GDM) is a specific type of diabetes that occurs during pregnancy. This condition differs from either type 1 or type 2 diabetes in that it develops during pregnancy and resolves after the baby is born. Gestational diabetes occurs when your body is unable to process sugar appropriately and you develop abnormally high levels of glucose in the bloodstream. Your body naturally creates insulin to utilize glucose that enters the bloodstream after eating. For some women, pregnancy causes changes in their bodies so that they do not make enough insulin, or that the insulin that they do make is no longer effective.

Your body normally uses glucose for energy, but if it stays in the bloodstream, the cells cannot use it. This can cause you to feel tired and can result in damage to your circulation and internal organs. It can also affect how your baby grows, as well as his overall health. You may also be at higher risk of developing type 2 diabetes later in life if you are diagnosed with gestational diabetes. To better understand how to care for yourself during pregnancy and to protect against GDM, it is important to know your level of risk for this condition as well as how gestational diabetes will be treated if you are diagnosed.

RISK FACTORS FOR GESTATIONAL DIABETES

There are some risk factors that may increase your chances of developing gestational diabetes with pregnancy. A risk factor is something that increases the possibility that you will contract a certain condition. Some factors are common to more than one illness, so having these factors as part of your life may predispose you to other types of illnesses as well.

Some risk factors can be changed; these are also called modifiable risk factors, but others are beyond your control.

WEIGHT GAIN DURING PREGNANCY

Your weight is one of the most important risk factors associated with gestational diabetes. How much you weigh, how your weight is distributed on your body, and how much you have gained during pregnancy can all impact your diabetes risk. It is normal and healthy to gain some weight during pregnancy, but if weight gain is not managed well, you can put yourself at higher risk of health problems.

If you were overweight or obese before becoming pregnant, you may increase your chances of developing gestational diabetes. Being overweight affects how your body uses insulin to control blood glucose levels and you may be more likely to have difficulty with unstable blood sugar. Many people who are overweight eat foods that contribute to weight gain or an inability to lose weight effectively, especially increased amounts of carbohydrates and fats. Increased intake of refined carbohydrates can cause your blood sugar levels to climb very high, and the body needs to respond by secreting more insulin. Once insulin takes care of the excess glucose in the bloodstream, your levels may return to normal, but by repeating this pattern, your body may become less effective at controlling your blood sugar. Additionally, if you have excess blood glucose, insulin will use this sugar for energy, rather than using stored fat. Ultimately, this makes it very difficult to lose weight.

Although it is normal to gain weight during pregnancy, if you have gained a significant amount of weight, especially in the first trimester, you may also be putting yourself at risk of developing gestational diabetes. A 2010 study performed by Kaiser Permanente found that women who gained significant amounts of weight during their first trimesters were more likely to develop gestational diabetes during their second and third trimesters when compared with women who did not gain too much weight during the first few weeks of pregnancy. The exact reasons for this are not entirely clear, but experts believe that putting on excessive weight quickly during the first several weeks of pregnancy can cause insulin resistance and can slow down the abilities of the pancreas to secrete adequate amounts of insulin.

Your health care provider should give you guidelines for how much weight you should gain during pregnancy. These guidelines are based on your body mass index (BMI) at the start of your pregnancy and they are recommended by the Institute of Medicine. If you were underweight or had a healthy BMI before pregnancy, you may need to gain more weight than if you had a higher BMI before pregnancy. If you gain a significant amount of weight above the recommendation, even if you were at a normal weight before pregnancy, you can still increase your risk of gestational diabetes.

METABOLIC SYNDROME
Some people have a condition known as metabolic syndrome, which is a group of factors that not only can raise your risk of gestational diabetes, but may lead to other conditions as well, such as heart disease. It is called metabolic syndrome because it affects body processes to increase the risk for certain illnesses, and it is a collection of several different situations that pose as risk factors. You may be considered to have metabolic syndrome if you have at least three of these factors together:

- *Being overweight and carrying excess weight around your middle.* This shape differs slightly from women who carry extra weight on the hips or thighs and may be referred to as an "apple" shape. Carrying more weight around the waist before you became pregnant can increase your risk of certain illnesses, such as heart disease and diabetes.

- *Having difficulties controlling blood glucose levels.* If you have been told that you have prediabetes or insulin resistance, you may have another factor that contributes to metabolic syndrome. Difficulties with controlling your blood sugar levels and insulin resistance from the body's cells can cause difficulties with regular maintenance of blood glucose.
- *Hypertension.* Having high blood pressure can be dangerous during pregnancy because it impacts blood flow to your baby. It can also increase your health problems and your risk of having difficulties during delivery. Having high blood pressure is another factor associated with metabolic syndrome.
- *High triglycerides and LDL cholesterol.* Triglycerides are a type of fat that is in the bloodstream. They are created from excess calories that haven't otherwise been used for energy. Too many triglycerides circulating through the bloodstream can lead to heart disease. LDL is the "bad" cholesterol that also contributes to heart disease and hardening of the arteries. This condition can impact your circulation, which not only adds to the negative effects of high blood sugar, but also further increases your risk of heart attack or stroke.
- *Low levels of HDL cholesterol.* Also known as the "good" cholesterol, HDL is responsible for getting rid of excess amounts of LDL cholesterol that is associated with heart disease.

According to the National Heart, Lung, and Blood Institute, your risk of developing diabetes is five times greater if you have metabolic syndrome when compared with someone who does not have it. You can control whether you develop metabolic syndrome by managing your weight, your blood pressure, and your cholesterol levels, which will also further reduce your risk of developing gestational diabetes.

PHYSICAL ACTIVITY
Along the lines of weight control is how much exercise you get on a weekly basis. Your levels of physical activity can have an impact on your risk of gestational diabetes. Exercise is so important for your circulation, strengthening the heart and making it more efficient, improving your flexibility and muscle tone, and managing your blood glucose levels.

Regular exercise is beneficial to everyone, and the Centers for Disease Control and Prevention recommend that all adults get at least 150 minutes of moderate-intensity exercise each week. Moderate-intensity means that you break a sweat and it may be a little difficult to carry a conversation because you are breathing harder. Exercise is especially beneficial if you have weight to lose as well. Exercise requires you to use your muscles, which causes the heart to beat faster to continue to supply enough oxygenated blood. This increased work boosts your metabolism, or how quickly you burn calories. If you exercise regularly, you may be more likely to burn calories more quickly and less likely to store excess fat. When paired with a healthy diet, this can help you to lose weight at a faster pace and can reduce your risk of gestational diabetes.

DIET AND NUTRITION
What you eat, as well as the types of foods that you eat, can all impact your risk of developing GDM if you are pregnant. Your food intake has a direct impact on your blood sugar levels, and

if you eat large amounts of foods that cause high blood glucose, you could be at risk. Almost all foods are classified as proteins, fats, carbohydrates, or a combination of these three. Each of these types of nutrients are broken down in the body during digestion, and carbohydrates tend to have the most rapid results. Refined carbohydrates, in particular, can make your blood sugar rise so quickly that your pancreas will be scrambling to secrete enough insulin to counteract the situation. Some examples of refined carbohydrates include white sugar, syrup, white flour, fruit juice, dried fruits, and many desserts and sweets.

If your diet contains large amounts of foods that are high in sweets and refined carbohydrates, you may be causing erratic spikes in blood sugar when you eat. After a while, your body may be more likely to have difficulties with controlling your blood glucose levels and your pancreas may not be able to keep up with producing insulin in response. Alternatively, the cells may become resistant to the insulin secreted, resulting in consistently high blood glucose levels and the possibility of gestational diabetes.

STRESS AND DEPRESSION

Stress and depression also play a role in your risk of developing GDM. Stress management may not be easy, especially while pregnant, but learning to control how stress affects you and taking steps to manage depression can help to change your risk of diabetes. Stress can have an impact on your blood glucose levels, as continued amounts of stress cause your blood glucose to rise. Over time, you may have a hard time keeping your blood sugar within a normal range.

Additionally, depression contributes to your risk of gestational diabetes. When you suffer from depression, you may be less likely to perform routine tasks to take care of yourself. You may also feel more of a desire for "comfort" foods: those foods that make you feel better while eating but that can wreak havoc on your blood glucose. Depression may be categorized depending on your symptoms and the length of time that you have been having them. If you have feelings of hopelessness, guilt, worthlessness, sadness, or diminished energy; or if you have had difficulty concentrating, have had sleep problems, or a general loss of interest in your usual activities for a period of more than two weeks, talk with your health care provider. These feelings may not go away on their own and it is important to control your feelings of stress or depression for the health of yourself and your baby.

FACTORS OUTSIDE OF YOUR CONTROL
Beyond weight control, exercise, and nutrition, there are other risk factors, although they may be beyond your control. One factor that you cannot change is your ethnic background. There are some groups of women who are more likely to develop GDM because of their race, as the condition tends to occur more commonly within certain people groups. For some reason, women who are Hispanic or Native American tend to be more likely to develop GDM than women of other backgrounds. Additionally, women who have a first-degree relative with diabetes may be more likely to develop gestational diabetes during pregnancy. For example, if your father has type 2 diabetes, you may be at higher risk of developing gestational diabetes.

THE IMPACT OF DIABETES ON OTHERS

Gestational diabetes is not only problematic for you, but it can also have a negative impact on your baby. A baby who is born to a mother who has GDM may be more likely to have a large body weight. This is particularly true if the mother did not control her blood glucose levels very well during pregnancy.

Because the baby takes in nutrients and glucose from the mother through the placenta, excess glucose in the bloodstream can cross the placenta, telling the baby's body to produce more insulin to manage it. Over time, this can cause the baby to grow to be large in size, in a condition known as macrosomia. Macrosomia is defined as a birth weight of greater than 8 lb., 13 oz., or 4,000 gm.

Having a very large baby at birth also puts you and the baby at higher risks of complications during delivery. It can be difficult to deliver a baby of average size, but trying to deliver a large baby can cause complications such as excessive blood loss, tearing of the vaginal tissues, or injuries to the baby during birth, such as shoulder dystocia, broken collarbone, or the need for forceps or vacuum extraction. Many women who have babies born with macrosomia require cesarean sections to avoid some of the risk of birth injuries.

Babies born to mothers who had poorly controlled blood glucose levels during pregnancy may also be at risk of having low blood sugar after delivery. Before birth, the infant receives a regular amount of glucose from the mother, a condition that quickly changes following delivery. If the infant does not eat right away, he may have a drop in blood glucose levels, causing hypoglycemia. Often, babies born to mothers with gestational diabetes must have their blood sugar levels checked closely for the first day after birth. Other risks that may also occur include larger-than-normal organs, poor suck reflex and poor feeding ability after birth, floppy muscle tone, and an increased risk of jaundice. Additionally, infants born to mothers with poorly controlled blood glucose levels are more likely to struggle with being overweight or obese later in life.

Beyond potential complications for yourself and your baby, gestational diabetes can also cause problems with future pregnancies if you decide to have another baby. It can also cause further health issues down the road, including an increased risk of developing type 2 diabetes.

If you have gestational diabetes with your current pregnancy, you are more likely to develop the condition again with subsequent pregnancies. Having GDM during pregnancy can take its toll on the body, and you may need to carefully consider when or if you want to have another child, in order to allow yourself time to heal. If you do become pregnant again after having GDM, you may need to check your blood glucose levels more frequently during your next pregnancy, as well as continue to follow a healthy diet and get regular exercise.

Having GDM increases your risk of developing type 2 diabetes later. Although gestational diabetes should resolve after you have delivered your baby, type 2 diabetes can be a life-long condition in which you must manage your blood sugar, diet, and activity levels. The National Diabetes Education Program states that women who had GDM during pregnancy are seven times more likely to develop type 2 diabetes when compared with those who did not have gestational diabetes. You have up to a 60 percent chance of developing type 2 diabetes in the next 10 to 20 years if you have had GDM.

Despite the risks and complications associated with GDM, there are steps that you can take to protect yourself from developing the condition. One of the most important processes in diagnosing gestational diabetes is detection. You can work with your health care provider during your prenatal check ups to be tested for gestational diabetes. Understanding what detection methods are available, as well as what to do if you are diagnosed, are important steps toward managing your health during pregnancy.

DETECTING GESTATIONAL DIABETES

Detection methods for screening and testing for gestational diabetes should ideally begin with your first prenatal visit. If you have risk factors, your doctor may want to perform some initial testing at your first visit. If your test results show that you do not have gestational diabetes, you will then need to be tested again later in pregnancy, preferably between the 24th and 28th week of gestation. If you do not have a high risk of gestational diabetes, you should still be tested mid-way through your pregnancy.

SCREENING VS. TESTING

When considering detection of gestational diabetes, it is important to first understand the difference between screening and testing for the disease. Screening is a process that is performed on a larger number of people who are within a population at risk of developing a certain condition. For example, screening for gestational diabetes is typically performed on all pregnant women at a certain point during pregnancy because the condition develops within this population. Alternatively, screening for gestational diabetes is obviously not performed among men or women who are not pregnant, although this population may represent another at-risk group for screening of a different disease, such as type 2 diabetes.

There are many benefits to the screening process. First, experts recognize that there are certain illnesses present in some groups in the community. Second, screening is often done when no symptoms are present. You may have a screening test done even if you feel fine or have no symptoms of the disease for which you are being screened. Because the screening is often done at an early time in which you may not have symptoms, the disease can be detected earlier than if you waited to actually develop the symptoms. In this manner, early detection through screening provides the benefit of "catching" the disease before symptoms start or you develop complications. This is also beneficial from a financial perspective, because it is easier to screen a larger number of people for a condition and then treat the few who have it when compared to only providing treatment after symptoms and complications have developed. Often the complications are quite costly, both in terms of financial as well as personal expense.

In contrast, diagnostic testing is done then to provide a diagnosis if you do not pass a screening exam. You may have a routine screening exam that would normally be performed on all pregnant patients, even if you do not have symptoms. If the screening results show that you might have the disease, you can then undergo testing to diagnose the condition and start treatment, if necessary. Some patients who are already at high risk of developing certain conditions may bypass the screening procedures and simply undergo diagnostic testing anyway.

In the case of gestational diabetes, your health care provider may offer some tests to screen you for the condition because you are pregnant and if you do not pass the screening tests, you will be referred for other diagnostic testing. Alternatively, if you were to develop symptoms of gestational diabetes before you went through screening, or if you are already at high risk, you may forego the official screening and simply have the diagnostic testing instead. There are a number of tests that can be performed as part of the detection process for gestational diabetes. Some of these tests are used as screening tests and some are done for diagnosing the condition. Which test your health care provider orders may depend on your condition and your risks of having gestational diabetes.

The fasting glucose test is a relatively routine test that can provide a snapshot of what your glucose levels are at one point in time. The test requires a blood sample, which may be obtained by either taking a small sample from a vein in the arm or by pricking the end of your finger. Before taking this test, you must go without eating for a certain period of time, usually about 8 hours.

Normally, your blood glucose levels should be relatively low because you have not been digesting food for several hours and therefore not contributing glucose to the bloodstream. After your last meal, your body should have secreted insulin to get the glucose from the bloodstream into the cells. By the time you have fasted for several hours, you may feel tired and hungry because your cells need energy.

If the fasting glucose test shows that you still have a significant amount of glucose in your bloodstream, the health care provider knows that your body may not be processing glucose as effectively as it should. While a fasting glucose is often done in the morning after you haven't eaten overnight, you may also have a random blood glucose test, which checks your blood sugar at any time of day, whether or not you have fasted. If you have a random glucose test, you will need to tell your doctor the time that you last ate and perhaps what you had to eat. This can give your doctor a better idea of what your blood glucose results might be and how they will be affected.

The fasting glucose test can be performed as a screening tool or as a diagnostic test. Whether or not you will need more testing depends on your results and what other tests have already been performed. The test measures the amount of glucose in your blood and is read as milligrams of blood glucose per deciliter of blood (mg/dL). A normal fasting blood glucose result is between 70 and 100 mg/dL. If your result is between 100 and 125 mg/dL, you may be classified as having a condition known as impaired glucose tolerance, in which your body has trouble processing glucose in a timely manner. When screening for GDM, a result between 100 and 125 mg/dL warrants further testing to confirm a diagnosis.

If your fasting glucose test results are 126 mg/dL or more, your doctor should do more tests to further confirm that you have gestational diabetes. Again, you may need more testing at this point to determine if your body continues to respond in this manner. For instance, a second fasting glucose test may be ordered for another day, and if that result is also high, it represents a pattern of problems with processing glucose in your body. Whether or not you have another fasting glucose test or another diagnostic test on a different day will also depend on your initial result. If your fasting glucose result was very high, your doctor may already confirm that you have gestational diabetes.

The fasting glucose test is just one test that may point to a diagnosis of GDM, whether it is done to screen for the condition or to confirm its presence. Another type of test, the oral glucose tolerance test, is a common screening tool used among pregnant women to look for signs of impaired glucose tolerance.

THE ORAL GLUCOSE TOLERANCE TEST

The oral glucose tolerance test (OGTT) determines how well your body processes glucose for a period of time after you take in a certain amount of glucose through a type of drink. The OGTT may be used as a testing measure midway through your pregnancy if you do not have a high risk of gestational diabetes. Unless you have no risk factors, your doctor should order the OGTT for you at a point a little over halfway through your pregnancy (around 24-28 weeks). The OGTT may also be performed if you have had other testing done, such as a fasting glucose test, in order to confirm whether you have gestational diabetes.

You can prepare for the test by eating a well-rounded diet that has a balance of carbohydrates, proteins, and fats. This is not the time to limit your carbohydrate intake, however, you also do not want to go overboard and eat too many either. You can keep a balance of carbohydrates in your diet by eating approximately 150 g per day for several days leading up to the test, in addition to adding some foods that contain protein and fat. You may also want to avoid exercising or smoking for a day before your test. Some medications, such as corticosteroids or blood pressure medications can also impact the outcome of your test. Talk with your health care provider to review all of the medications you are currently taking and to discuss any restrictions that may be necessary. Your provider may decide that you need to temporarily stop taking certain medications before your test.

Before the test, you will be instructed to fast for at least 8 hours. This test is often scheduled in the morning at many doctor's offices: having it done in the morning means that you can go without eating overnight and skip breakfast before going in to have your test. This saves you from going through a whole day without eating in order to have the test in the afternoon.

When you arrive for the test, you will have blood taken to check your glucose levels. This is a fasting blood glucose test, and the result will be used as a baseline for comparison. If your health care provider knows what your blood sugar levels are after fasting for 8 hours, he can then compare this level to results that will be taken after you have more glucose in your system later. You will need to have blood drawn for your initial fasting glucose test and for the follow up tests that will come later. This blood is checked either by taking it from a vein in your arm or through a finger stick.

Once you have had the fasting level drawn, you will then be instructed to drink a glucose drink that contains 75 g of glucose in it; this liquid is sometimes called glucola. It is very sweet, and some women have compared it to drinking sugary syrup of jellybeans. It comes in a variety of flavors; the most common is orange, although it may also taste like lemon-lime, fruit punch, grape, cherry, or cola. The drink may be given to you cold, which typically makes it taste a little better. Each doctor's office will have different policies in place about drinking the glucose solution, but most have a time limit for how long you can take to drink it. You may have between 5 and 10 minutes to drink the full amount; depending on the brand, it is 8 or 10 oz. per serving. Try to drink it quickly, instead of sipping it, even if you don't like the taste. Do your best not to think about the taste and instead focus on your health by drinking it. It is better to drink it relatively quickly and get it done so that you can go on to complete your testing.

After you drink the glucose beverage, you will need to wait to have your blood drawn. In fact, your blood will be drawn several times, typically at intervals of one hours and two hours after the drink. Depending on your glucose levels or the protocol at your provider's office, you may need a third blood test three hours after the drink as well. While waiting to have your blood drawn, you should relax and do a quiet activity. You will be asked to wait at the office during the test, so be prepared to stay and keep yourself occupied. You will not be allowed to eat anything during this time, but you may be allowed to drink water. Bring comfortable clothes that you can relax in while waiting, as well as another activity that is quiet but that will keep you busy, such as a book or magazine, puzzles, or journaling. Since you may be waiting at least 2 hours, plan ahead by bringing something to do to help pass the time.

When the first blood test is done, the results will show your blood glucose levels approximately one hour after your glucose drink. This result gives your provider a good idea of how your body is responding to a large influx of glucose. At the 2-hour mark, the levels again will show how your body is responding to the glucose, only this time, it has had even more time to process the large amount of sugar. By two hours, your glucose levels should be lower than your 1-hour level, which shows that your body is consistently processing glucose over time.

A normal result for an OGTT is provided in a range of outcomes and like the fasting glucose test, is expressed in milligrams of glucose per deciliter of blood (mg/dL). For most laboratories processing the blood sample, the normal outcome for the fasting glucose level before the OGTT should be less than 95 mg/dL. After one hour, the normal level should be less than 180 mg/dL. After two hours, your blood glucose should be less than 153 mg/dL. Your health care provider may also give you a reference range for what outcome he or she expects your blood glucose to be at certain points during the test based on the lab's machinery.

If your glucose levels are between 140 and 200 mg/dL after 2 hours, you may have impaired glucose tolerance, also called prediabetes. This is very important to know because it can lead to diabetes. You may need further testing to rule out a diabetes diagnosis or you may need to check your blood sugar levels more frequently during your pregnancy. If your blood glucose is still over 200 mg/dL after 2 hours, you most likely have gestational diabetes. However, this should be confirmed with a second test on another day for diabetes in order for your provider to give you an actual diagnosis. Your doctor may ask you to return for another fasting glucose test or a second oral glucose tolerance test a few days after your first in order to compare the results. If your results are still high after the second test, then your provider can confirm a diagnosis. If your 2-hour result is significantly over 200 mg/dL during your first OGTT, your physician may opt for treatment right away in order to protect your health and that of your baby, such as by prescribing a dose of insulin to bring your blood glucose levels back to normal. You will then need to further discuss a schedule of checking your glucose levels and what types of management techniques you will need to do to keep your blood sugar within a normal range.

THE HEMOGLOBIN A1C TEST
Also called the glycated hemoglobin test, the hemoglobin A1C is another type of test that may be part of monitoring of blood glucose. The hemoglobin A1C is a blood test, but instead of checking what your blood glucose levels are in the moment, it determines what your levels have been for the past several weeks. This is done by checking the red blood cells.

There are several types of blood cells, and each have their different functions. The red blood cells are responsible for circulating through the bloodstream to carry oxygen to the tissues and organs. Each red blood cell has a hemoglobin molecule attached to it. Hemoglobin is a protein that carries oxygen. When glucose levels in the bloodstream are elevated, the hemoglobin molecules essentially become coated with glucose, also known as being glycated. Once glucose binds to the hemoglobin molecule, it stays there for the life of the cell. Because red blood cells have a lifespan of about 120 days, this test can tell your doctor how much glucose has been attached to the hemoglobin for that time, essentially giving an idea of what your blood glucose levels have been for the past 3 to 4 months.

The hemoglobin A1C test may be performed during an initial visit to the doctor after you determine that you are pregnant. In some cases, having this test may show that you had diabetes before becoming pregnant. If your result of the hemoglobin A1C is higher than normal or you have other factors that put you at high risk of gestational diabetes, you will then need further testing, such as through the oral glucose tolerance test. If you have been diagnosed with gestational diabetes, you may need to have the hemoglobin A1C performed again in during your pregnancy to determine your average levels of glucose over a period of time.

There are usually not any restrictions before undergoing the hemoglobin A1C. Because the test looks at glucose over time, fasting or avoiding certain activities a few hours or days before the test will have no impact on the results. It is a blood test, so you may need to have it done at your doctor's office or in a lab. To get the sample, blood is usually collected from a vein in your arm.

The hemoglobin A1C results are expressed as a percentage. This percentage is the amount of hemoglobin that is coated with glucose. The higher the percentage, the larger amount of hemoglobin that is glycated. Among people who do not have diabetes, a normal hemoglobin A1C level is about 5.7 percent. A diagnosis of prediabetes, or impaired glucose tolerance, occurs when the hemoglobin A1C level is between 5.7 and 6.4 percent. A person with a hemoglobin A1C level above 6.5 percent will most likely be diagnosed with diabetes.

GLUCOSE MONITORING

If you are at high risk of gestational diabetes or you have been diagnosed with the condition, you will need to check your blood glucose on a regular basis to ensure that it remains within a normal range. Your doctor can give you a range of normal limits for what your blood glucose levels should be. You may be able to control your glucose by making dietary changes, or you may need to start taking medications. How you manage your glucose first depends on the results that you get when you test at home. There are several methods of testing your blood sugar after you have been diagnosed with gestational diabetes.

When you get ready to start testing your blood sugar on your own at home, you will need to gather the right supplies. Most people check their blood sugar by a finger stick. This involves using a lancet, which is a small instrument with a sharp end that pricks the skin of the finger and allows you to squeeze out a drop of blood. You do not need to try to obtain any more blood than this at a time; only a drop is usually needed for each test. Glucose testing strips look like small strips of paper; the end of one of these strips is plugged into the glucose-testing monitor. When you have a drop of blood on your finger, you put it onto the end of the testing strip opposite of the other end that is in the glucose meter. The meter will read the amount of glucose that is within that drop of blood. After several seconds, the meter will give a result, expressed as a number, and that is your blood glucose level. When you first have to check your glucose on your own, your nurse may help you learn how to use the equipment until you are comfortable.

Your doctor will also give you a schedule as to how often and at what times of day you should check your glucose. You may need to test before meals or after waking up. Some women also need to test their blood sugar after they have exercised or if they are sick, as these situations can also cause a change in blood sugar. In addition to knowing when to check your glucose, you should also know what the ideal results should be. For instance, you can expect that if you are hungry and getting ready to eat, your blood sugar would be lower than if you checked it 30 minutes after eating a meal. If your blood sugar levels are consistently high, you may need orders from your doctor about what to do if you cannot control your glucose with a proper diet.

Health care providers have a slight range of what they consider to be normal limits for glucose results, depending on when you check your blood sugar. If you check your glucose just after waking up or before eating, it should be approximately 95 mg/dL or less. If you check again an hour after a meal, a normal level should be less than 140 mg/dL. You can record your blood glucose results to give to your doctor so he or she can determine how well you are able to control your levels. You may also need to record what foods and how much of each type you eat each day. Your doctor or dietitian can then compare your intake with your glucose results. If you are unable to manage your blood sugar through diet alone, your doctor may then decide that medication is necessary.

In some cases, you could be at risk of too low of blood sugar levels, also called hypoglycemia. It may be more likely to occur if you haven't eaten in a while or if you have done some activity that would require excess energy, such as exercising. If you develop hypoglycemia, you might feel shaky, irritable, or hungry; you might have difficulties concentrating or you might feel very tired. It is important to check your blood sugar if this occurs. If your glucose is very low when you test it, then you will need to eat or drink something to restore your blood sugar levels. When you receive directions from your doctor for managing high glucose levels, you should also have instructions for what to do if your blood sugar drops too low.

Another method of measuring glucose is through a continuous glucose monitor. This machine is a type of probe that measures glucose in the subcutaneous tissue on a regular basis, nearly eliminating the need for finger stick checks throughout the day. A sensor is inserted under the skin in an area with subcutaneous fat, such as the upper arm. The sensor reads glucose levels in the body on a regular basis and then transmits the information wirelessly to a machine that is worn on the body. The data is recorded in the machine, which allows you to find out what your current glucose is, as well as see how your glucose fluctuates throughout the day and night.

Continuous glucose monitoring methods are not always ordered for women who are pregnant. Although they provide a very regular recording of what your glucose levels are, there may be a slight lag in time and accuracy, since the probe is reading a result from subcutaneous tissue. Additionally, even with a monitor, you may still have to check your blood glucose at least once per day with a finger stick to determine how accurate the machine is and to calibrate it.

Alternatively, continuous glucose monitoring can be beneficial when you need to closely watch your glucose levels and check for results often. It can save you from repeatedly performing finger sticks to check your blood with a glucose meter. It also works well if you and your health care provider are trying to modify your regimen of managing your gestational diabetes;

for instance, if your doctor is trying to determine whether you need to add medication to your dietary regimen, he can look at the recordings of your glucose measurements and see trends over time.

Continuous glucose monitoring may or may not be covered by your insurance company. Your health care provider will determine if having this type of monitor is beneficial for you, and together you can weigh the advantages and disadvantages of using this type of system.

THE NON-STRESS TEST

If you are diagnosed with gestational diabetes, you might need more check ups with your physician and extra tests as well. Extra prenatal visits and testing are done to continue to monitor your health and that of your baby. Because gestational diabetes can cause complications with your own health or your baby's well being, you may need to have testing to ensure that he is healthy and growing well.

A non-stress test is a type of exam that can determine if your baby's heart rate is within the normal range. The test checks for when the baby moves, at which point the heart rate should increase. During the test, a nurse will place sensors on your abdomen at specific locations over where the baby is in your belly. These sensors are held in place by a belt and they are connected to a monitor. The sensors have dual purposes: if you have any contractions during the non-stress test, one of the sensors will pick up on this and record it. Contractions can affect the baby's heart rate. The other sensor picks up on the baby's heart rate during movement and records it on the monitor.

You will be given a device to signal when you feel the baby move. During the test, you will rest on a bed for about 30 minutes. Every time you feel the baby move or you feel a contraction; you push the device to record it. Later, the physician can check the recording and compare when you felt the baby move with his heart rate at that time. The baby's heart rate should increase during the times that you felt movement. The non-stress test may be done at your doctor's office or you may need to go to the hospital on an outpatient basis. This test may be done after you have reached at least 32 weeks' gestation if you are taking insulin to manage your gestational diabetes, or closer to your delivery date if you have GDM that is managed through diet but not medication.

Another test, called the biophysical profile (BPP), involves a non-stress test but also includes an ultrasound that is performed at the same time. This test is also done to measure how healthy your baby is and may also be performed if there are more conclusive issues with your pregnancy; for instance, if you also have high blood pressure or if your baby is not growing well. It is most often done during your third trimester, typically after at least 32 weeks' gestation.

The BPP determines the overall health of your baby by checking several signs that he is growing and has normal vital signs. Depending on the state of your own health, you may need more than one biophysical profile test. The main items that this test checks for are your baby's heart rate with movement, breathing patterns, muscle tone, movement, and the amount of amniotic fluid present.

There are not too many restrictions that you will need to follow before having this test, but your doctor may require that you have a full bladder before starting. If so, you may need to drink several glasses of water and then wait a few minutes before the test gets underway. If you smoke or are taking special medications during your pregnancy, talk with your health care provider about stopping before having this test. Like the non-stress test, you may be able to have the BPP done at your doctor's office if they have the capabilities, or you may need to have the test done at a hospital.

The biophysical profile (BPP) starts with a non-stress test as described above. This test takes about 30 minutes and records your baby's heart rate during movement or if you have any contractions. Additionally, you will also have an abdominal ultrasound as part of the BPP. During the ultrasound, the technologist will expose your belly and put a cool gel on the skin. She uses a transducer, which bounces sound waves to the internal structures of your abdomen and pelvis, and then transmits the images onto a monitor. This is how you are able to see a type of picture of your baby. The technologist is able to view the baby, see him move, and take measurements if necessary. The ultrasound may take another 30 minutes.

The results of the BPP are documented as a type of score, based on the measurements the test is intended for: heart rate with movement (the non-stress test), muscle tone, body movement, breathing, and amniotic fluid. Your health care provider may review the parameters of what is considered normal with the biophysical profile results. Typically during the non-stress test, the baby's heart rate should increase by at least 15 beats per minute with movement or contractions. During a 30-minute non-stress test, you can expect to have at least 2 episodes of an increase in the baby's heart rate with movement, although this result can vary.

The baby's muscle tone is checked through the ultrasound. The technologist can evaluate this by seeing if the baby moves his arms and legs, flexes his extremities, or generates some other form of movement using the muscles. This part of the test also determines that the baby is in the appropriate position in the uterus, which is typically with the arms and legs flexed and the head tucked toward the chest.

Body movement is also determined by the ultrasound, but when you have the non-stress test, you may also signify when you feel the baby move. You can expect that the baby should move at least three times throughout the course of the entire test, including the non-stress test and the ultrasound. This movement includes moving just the arms or legs, as well as the whole body.

Although a baby does not breathe air until after he is born, he will still have a breathing pattern in the womb. This is the baby's practice at breathing, even though his lungs are not fully mature. During the biophysical profile test, you can expect to see the baby practice at breathing at least once, which should last a minimum of 30 seconds. Finally, during the ultrasound, the technologist can determine and measure how much amniotic fluid is present around the baby. There should be at least a pocket of fluid that can be measured and your doctor will determine if this is enough, not enough, or too much fluid.

The BPP is scored with a point system, with 2 points given for a normal response in each of the five sections. If there is an abnormal outcome in a particular area, that section is given 0 points. The biophysical profile is then given a result as a number between 0 and 10, with 8 to10 points being the best outcome and signifying a healthy baby. If you have a result of less than 8, you may need to have another BPP at a later time to determine if you would have similar results or if the baby has different behavior on another day. If your BPP result is less than 4 points, you may need to have further testing, such as laboratory studies, a test of amniotic fluid, or other ultrasounds, to better determine the health of your baby.

During the test, you will have to lie on your back, both for the non-stress test and the abdominal ultrasound. If you have a full bladder for the test, you may become quite uncomfortable by the time the test is over. It may also be difficult to lie flat on your back, particularly if you are close to your due date. Notify your doctor or the technologist doing the test if you are particularly uncomfortable.

It's natural to feel nervous about the results of a non-stress test or biophysical profile. There may be a lot of activity from the nurses, the doctor, or the technician who are all trying to get you settled and ready. It can be hard not to worry about the results and what they mean and you may have a lot of questions during the test. In most cases, if a technologist is performing your ultrasound, he or she cannot answer many questions, especially if they are related to the baby's outcome. You may have to wait through the test and talk with your doctor about the results.

OTHER BASICS OF TESTING

Testing for gestational diabetes may be done if you are classified as a high-risk patient for developing the condition, or if you went through a screening procedure that showed you could benefit from further testing. Because GDM often shows up during pregnancy at or around a similar time for many women, there is a certain timeline that many doctor's offices follow when going through the screening and testing process for their patients.

Unless you are at high risk of developing gestational diabetes and this information is obvious and available to the health care provider at your first prenatal visit, you may only go through screening procedures at approximately halfway through your pregnancy. This is because most women who develop GDM do so during the second and third trimester. If you were diagnosed with gestational diabetes during your first trimester, there may be a chance that you already had diabetes before you became pregnant.

Gestational diabetes tends to occur later in pregnancy because of the effects of hormones from the placenta. The placenta normally provides nutrients to the baby that come from the mother. Sometimes during pregnancy, a woman must make larger amounts of insulin to keep up with excess glucose in the bloodstream. During the second trimester and later, the placenta starts producing more hormones that somehow interfere with how insulin is used in the mother's body in some women. This is how gestational diabetes develops. The condition ends when the baby is delivered because the placenta is also delivered at that time and the hormones are no longer in the body.

Because doctors know that gestational diabetes shows up later in pregnancy, you will not be screened for it until later as well. This saves you from having multiple tests performed, such as undergoing a blood test early in pregnancy and then repeating it again several months later. Additionally, the blood glucose problems that develop with GDM will most likely not be present early in pregnancy, so there is little point in performing testing during the first trimester. Again, this is only if you are not classified as being high risk for the condition, which otherwise might warrant earlier testing for diabetes or impaired glucose tolerance.

If you are seeking care from a physician or midwife who performs glucose screenings as part of prenatal visits, you usually do not have much of a choice about when the screenings are done. You may schedule your test for certain times, but it is typically done between 24 and 28 weeks' gestation. It is important to follow through with testing during this time to ensure that changes haven't occurred in your blood glucose levels since you became pregnant. At this time, the main test that will be performed is the oral glucose tolerance test, however, many doctor's offices have their own protocols, and some may use a different test first. This depends on your history and risk factors.

At your first prenatal visit, you can expect to go through a screening process for your risks of diabetes, in addition to other exams that you will need, such as your vital signs, height, and weight. Your health care provider should assess your BMI and your vital signs, including heart rate, respiratory rate, and blood pressure. Your provider should also take a thorough history to assess if you have any risks associated with diabetes, including whether you have had gestational diabetes with a previous pregnancy, if you have ever had a baby who was larger than 9 lbs. at birth, if you have any first-degree relatives with diabetes, or whether you need to take any medications to maintain normal blood sugar levels. Finally, your provider should also be aware of any other health conditions you may have that can affect your pregnancy, such as high blood pressure, high cholesterol, thyroid disease, or polycystic ovary disease.

During your prenatal visits, your doctor should give you plenty of information about how to keep yourself healthy, whether or not you are eventually diagnosed with gestational diabetes. You may receive counseling and information about good nutrition, how to manage your weight and what your goals for weight gain should be, what supplements or vitamins may be necessary, possible risks of depression or mental health issues, what immunizations you might need, and how to increase your physical activity.

Your doctor should also provide information about the risks associated with GDM and explain the purpose of testing. If you are diagnosed with gestational diabetes, your doctor should let you know what further tests you will need to maintain control of your health, such as by coming up with a schedule for checking your glucose on a regular basis or taking certain medications to control your blood sugar. If possible, a referral to a dietitian or diabetes educator can be helpful to assist you with planning a diet that can keep your blood sugar levels stable.

Your baby will also need to be monitored more closely if you have been diagnosed with GDM. Your provider should give you an idea of any additional tests that may need to be done to check the health of your baby, such as extra ultrasounds, a check of amniotic fluid, a non-stress test, or a biophysical profile. Many women who consistently maintain normal blood glucose levels despite having gestational diabetes can go on to have healthy pregnancies with few complications. By working with your health care provider to undergo testing for this condition and to cooperate through treatment, you can stay healthy and have a successful delivery.

Treatment of Gestational Diabetes

A diagnosis of gestational diabetes requires a number of interventions that can help to keep blood glucose levels within a normal range and prevent complications associated with uncontrolled hyperglycemia, which occurs when blood glucose runs too high. Understanding the potential risks to the mother's health and that of the baby when GDM is not managed well often helps many women to take the necessary steps to take charge of their health after being diagnosed.

There are several different treatment options available for management of GDM. Some of these options involve short-term management of the current situation, while others may be long-term.

After diagnosis, your health care provider may refer you to a diabetes educator or a dietician to help you with the lifestyle changes necessary for controlling GDM. A diabetes educator can help you to gather the supplies you will need to check your own blood glucose levels, she can show you how to record and track your glucose results, and she will make sure you understand when to test your glucose and what to do if your blood sugar levels fall outside of the normal range. A dietician can help you plan a diet that will help to keep your blood sugar levels stable and avoid dramatic spikes or drops in blood glucose. A dietician or educator may also be able to help you come up with a system for implementing activity into your lifestyle, which may help you lose weight if you need to, but which can also provide a consistent level of physical fitness that will improve your circulation, strength, and flexibility, as well as help to control your blood sugar.

Making changes toward a healthy lifestyle involves long-term management of your diabetes. By eating right, exercising regularly, and making positive changes for your health, you can control your gestational diabetes. Even after delivery, if you no longer have GDM, you may still have great control of your health if you continue to maintain the changes you made during pregnancy.

When you are managing gestational diabetes, you will also need short-term solutions at times. For example, illness can impact your blood sugar, but if you plan ahead for a sick day, you will be better prepared to keep your glucose stable, even if you do not eat regularly or are otherwise ill. When you have a schedule for when you should check your blood sugar and what results are normal, you can have a better idea of if you are managing your glucose well. You should also have a good back up plan for if your blood sugar levels are too high; whether that means taking oral medications or insulin. Alternatively, you should have a plan in place for what to do if your blood glucose levels fall too low. You will need to know what types of food or drink to take that can quickly raise your blood sugar back up to a normal range. All of these plans are short-term solutions for managing your gestational diabetes, which you will learn after diagnosis if you continue to work with your health care provider, diabetes educator, or dietician.

ORAL MEDICATIONS
The use of oral medications may be an option for you if you have gestational diabetes, particularly if you find that your blood sugar is not well controlled through diet and exercise alone. Oral medications work by helping to get glucose levels as close to normal as possible, although they may not be an option for everyone. Talk with your health care provider about your options for using oral medications to control your gestational diabetes. The two most common types of oral

medications used among pregnant women with diabetes are glyburide and metformin.

Glyburide is an oral medication that may be ordered for controlling your blood sugar. Recent studies have shown it to be a safe form of treatment for pregnant women with diabetes. Glyburide may be just as effective as insulin in some cases when managing elevated blood glucose levels associated with diabetes. Glyburide works in a number of ways, including stimulating the pancreas to secrete more insulin when needed and increasing the receptiveness of the cells to insulin so that there is less insulin resistance.

If you are given a prescription for glyburide, you may need to take it more than once a day. You will need to take it on a regular basis in order for it to be effective. Glyburide should be taken before a meal; it is typically taken first thing in the morning, about 30 minutes before eating breakfast. If it is ordered to be taken twice a day, you may need to take it in the evening before a bedtime snack.

One of the most common side effects associated with glyburide is when it lowers your blood glucose by too much. This can cause hypoglycemia, which can make you feel tired, weak, dizzy, or irritable. Some people also complain of nausea, a headache, or diarrhea when using glyburide. The typical dose is between 2.5 and 7.5 mg, once or twice a day, which is taken in pill form.

Metformin, another type of medication that may be taken orally to control gestational diabetes, controls blood glucose by making the cells more receptive to insulin. Because it does not necessarily stimulate the body to create more insulin in response to elevated glucose levels, metformin has fewer side effects that cause hypoglycemia. Instead, when it causes the cells to become more receptive to the insulin that is available, they more readily take up excess glucose, thereby better controlling levels of blood sugar.

Metformin is taken as a pill and usually needs to be taken with food. It may be ordered to be used on its own or in a combination with other medications, including insulin. Like glyburide, metformin should be taken as ordered on a regular basis in order for it to be the most effective. Some people complain of an upset stomach when taking metformin, so it helps to take it with food. If your doctor orders for you to take metformin, you may start with a smaller dose initially, and then increase the amount until you are taking 2 to 3 pills per day. The typical dose of metformin ranges between 500 mg to 850 mg.

Oral agents can work very effectively in controlling blood glucose levels and can be safe to use during pregnancy when under the direction of your doctor.

INSULIN
Some women with GDM require supplemental insulin to control their blood sugar levels. Your doctor may order insulin for your treatment depending on your current state of health, your blood sugar levels over a period of time, or if your body has not responded to oral medications for diabetes treatment.

The insulin that is used today for diabetes management is a synthetic form created to perform the same work of the insulin that you secrete in your body. Insulin is normally created in and secreted by the pancreas in response to increased levels of blood glucose. When your body does not create enough insulin or it is ineffective, you may need to take supplemental insulin.

There are several different types of insulin available, and they vary based on when they start working, when they have reached their peak effectiveness, and how long they last. The time at which insulin starts working is called its onset; the time that it becomes most effective in the body is its peak, and length of time that it lasts is its duration. Insulin is classified according to these factors and the types vary between rapid acting, regular, intermediate, or long acting.

Insulin comes in a vial of solution that must be drawn up with a needle and syringe. In addition to how quickly it acts and how long it lasts, it may have different strengths. It is important to follow your doctor's orders carefully to ensure that you are using the right type and strength of insulin that has been ordered for you.

Insulin is most often given by an injection; most people who need insulin must use a type of syringe and needle to inject the insulin into the subcutaneous fat, which is the fatty tissue found just underneath the skin. The most common sites for injection are the abdomen and the upper arm. Depending on the type of insulin you use, you may need to learn to draw it up with a needle and syringe and then give yourself an injection. The amount that you give is based on what your blood sugar levels are when you check them. Insulin may also be available in pen form, which is already drawn up into a syringe with a cartridge inside of it. When you need an injection, you dial in the prescribed amount and the pen sets itself to give the prescribed dose.

There are other methods of giving insulin, such as through an insulin pump attached to the body or through a port placed under the skin that makes administering insulin a little easier. For women with GDM, these may or may not be viable options, since the condition will resolve after delivery.

However, if you develop type 2 diabetes or your doctor feels that these methods of administration are appropriate for you during pregnancy, you may be able to take insulin this way.

After taking insulin, your blood sugar levels should go down. Managing blood sugar through insulin use should not only prevent you from having consistently high blood glucose levels, but should also prevent damage to your organs and circulation from chronically high blood sugar.

WEIGHT MANAGEMENT

Managing your weight is both a short- and long-term goal of treating gestational diabetes. Keeping your weight at a healthy level during your pregnancy can not only reduce your risk of developing gestational diabetes, but it can also make your pregnancy a little more comfortable if you are not carrying extra pounds.

Carrying a baby through pregnancy is not easy, and neither is losing weight, so this might be a lot to consider as far as your health is concerned. In fact, you should gain at least some weight during your pregnancy because the extra weight helps by nourishing your baby. Your baby, as well as the amniotic fluid, the extra fluid that develops in your circulatory system, and the placenta all add weight to your body, so you can expect your weight to go up.

Depending on your size before you became pregnant, you may need to gain more or less weight than someone else of a different size that is also pregnant. Your doctor should give you guidelines for how much weight you should gain, but if your BMI before pregnancy showed that you were either underweight or within a normal weight range, you can expect to gain between 25 to 40 pounds and still be healthy. If your

BMI before pregnancy showed that you were overweight or obese, you may need to gain only 15 to 25 pounds.

It may be difficult to control your weight during pregnancy, especially with food cravings and the need to eat extra calories every day. Although you are eating for two, you do not need to take in twice as many calories. However, you may need to increase your intake to between 350 and 500 extra calories per day while you are pregnant, depending on your weight. If you have been diagnosed with gestational diabetes, you can talk with a dietician or your health care provider to come up with a plan for eating and activity that can help you to safely gain an appropriate amount of weight while controlling your blood glucose. You may need to monitor and record your weight at home, and your weight will also be checked during prenatal visits.

If you were overweight before pregnancy and you are trying to manage your weight because you have gestational diabetes, there are still many things that you can do to protect your health. Talk with your doctor about how much weight to gain during your pregnancy. Although there are guidelines for weight gain depending on your BMI, your doctor may have slightly different recommendations for you. Although it may be tempting, avoid trying to go on a diet while you are pregnant. Diets, if they work, are only temporary solutions to a problem with weight and many people often gain the weight back. If you try to diet, you may also be missing some important nutrients that both you and your baby need.

Talk with your doctor about an exercise program that can help you to control your blood glucose level and that will be safe for you during pregnancy. It is important to attend all of your scheduled prenatal visits so that you can track your health and to have time to talk with your doctor about the best options for you to control your GDM by managing your weight.

It is important to attend all prenatal visits that you schedule so that you can continue to receive appropriate care during pregnancy. Your doctor will monitor your overall health and can talk with you about any issues or discomforts that you are having because of pregnancy. Prenatal visits are also a time to get ready for delivery. Your provider will monitor how the baby is growing, including approximating his size and weight, as well as what position he is in your belly. Additionally, because gestational diabetes can impact the baby's size and health, your delivery should be planned carefully to ensure that it is safe.

Depending on what is available at your provider's office, your prenatal visits may also be a time to review your diet and activity levels, or what medications or insulin you are taking. You may have an opportunity during this time to talk about any issues you are having with checking your blood glucose, using your equipment, or even just how diabetes has been making you feel while pregnant. You may receive further guidance if you need to make changes to your diet or your medication regimen.

In addition to monitoring and managing gestational diabetes, your prenatal visits are an important time where your doctor checks to determine that you are not developing any other health problems. You will have your blood pressure checked on a routine basis at these visits, as high blood pressure is a risk that can threaten a healthy pregnancy. Your doctor may also check other factors, such as whether you have fluid build up in your fingers or your lower legs, if you have had any vaginal spotting or bleeding, and your mental health and wellness, too.

If you develop other health problems during pregnancy or your blood glucose levels are difficult to control, your provider may order other tests that closely monitor your health and the health of your baby. These tests are sometimes beyond what must be done during a pregnancy that is not impacted by gestational diabetes, but in order to be safe, you may need to attend extra appointments to have these done.

TESTING AND APPOINTMENTS

Extra testing typically requires more appointments to be scheduled beyond your standard prenatal exams. Try not to worry if your doctor orders some extra tests. These are designed to monitor your health and check your baby's health as well, which is important. Try to think of extra testing as something that will guide you toward making the best decisions for your baby. If you do find that you might have pregnancy complications associated with gestational diabetes, you can follow your doctor's orders to take good care of yourself to protect your health as much as possible.

There are several different tests that may be necessary to check your baby's health if you have gestational diabetes. You probably had an ultrasound early in your pregnancy to confirm that you were pregnant and to check the heartbeat. An ultrasound may also be ordered later in pregnancy with GDM if your doctor wants to check your baby's well being. He or she may need to measure the size of your baby, check the location of the placenta, determine the amount of amniotic fluid, or see the position of your baby.

The non-stress test and biophysical profile test the overall health of your baby and these are often done among mothers with gestational diabetes to confirm the baby's health, due to the increased risk of complications. The non-stress test checks your baby's heart rate when he is moving around in the womb. The biophysical profile combines with the non-stress test to also check your baby's respiratory patterns, muscle movement, general movement, and the amount of amniotic fluid that is surrounding your baby.

An amniocentesis is a test that involves removing a small amount of amniotic fluid from the sac. The fluid is taken out through a needle that is inserted through your abdominal wall. The doctor will numb the area first where the needle will go in. Then, he uses an ultrasound to guide where to insert the needle so that he does not injure the baby. He collects a certain amount of fluid through the syringe and then removes the needle.

An amniocentesis may be performed if your doctor believes there is a risk to your baby because of a genetic or chromosomal abnormality. Sometimes, this test is also done if there is too much amniotic fluid surrounding the baby. This condition is called polyhydramnios, and it could possibly cause early labor, contribute to high blood pressure, or cause problems with the placenta. An amniocentesis may be performed to draw some of the extra fluid out of the amniotic sac and control polyhydramnios.

Your doctor will also monitor your baby and compare your health and the baby's health with your gestational age. Although typical length of gestation is 40 weeks, some women deliver before this and some women later, even up to 2 weeks beyond. With gestational diabetes, you may need to deliver at or before 40 weeks, depending on your baby's size and health. Some women must have their labor induced before 40 weeks to protect their bodies as well as their babies' health, in case the baby is growing too large. Induction occurs when the doctor gives you medications to start labor so that you can deliver your baby earlier than when you might have started laboring naturally. Before inducing labor, your doctor should test to determine if your baby is mature enough to come out and should determine the proper process of delivery, such as by a vaginal birth or C-section.

If you need specialized tests to check your baby's health or if your labor is induced early because of your gestational diabetes, you may need the help of some kinds of specialists who can care for you or your baby during this potentially stressful time.

WHEN TO SEE A SPECIALIST

There may come a time that you might need to see a specialist to help you with controlling your gestational diabetes and as someone who will direct your care through your pregnancy. A specialist may be someone who consults with your regular doctor about your care and provides guidance and direction. In some cases, a specialist may take over for your doctor entirely, for the remainder of your pregnancy. This would most likely occur if your condition becomes a high enough risk that your regular doctor or midwife would rather let you have the complete direction of someone who has had more experience with high-risk situations.

An endocrinologist is a medical doctor who specializes in conditions that affect the endocrine system, namely your hormones and metabolism. An endocrinologist may work as part of a team of doctors to direct your care, although some women with GDM do not work with an endocrinologist. Many endocrinologists work with patients who have type 1 or type 2 diabetes already, and can also help you manage your gestational diabetes. This specialist may provide direction for what your goal blood glucose levels should be, he or she may prescribe appropriate amounts of insulin or oral diabetes medications for you, and can help you monitor your weight. Some diabetes educators work in the offices of endocrinologists as resource personnel. These educators may help you find out where you can purchase diabetic supplies and can offer training for how to perform certain tasks.

A maternal-fetal specialist is a doctor with an obstetrics background who specifically works with pregnant women who are classified as being high risk. This type of doctor may also be called a perinatologist. The maternal-fetal specialist has typically had extra education beyond a standard OB/GYN and has a greater knowledge of potential complications that can occur during pregnancy, as well as how to treat them. He or she is also specially trained to perform certain procedures that can check the well being of your baby, such as amniocentesis. If you develop complications during your pregnancy, your regular OB/GYN doctor can consult with a maternal-fetal specialist for guidance, or the maternal-fetal specialist may become your primary doctor through the remainder of your pregnancy.

A neonatologist is a doctor who specializes in the care and treatment of newborn babies. This type of doctor may be asked to stand by during your delivery if your own doctor believes there is any risk to your baby. Many hospitals with neonatal intensive care units (NICUs) have neonatologists available so that if there are any complications during delivery, this type of specialist is immediately available. If your baby needs specialized care after delivery, such as help with breathing, assistance with feeding or controlling blood glucose levels, a neonatologist may assume care of your baby until he or she is ready to go home from the hospital. They may even be there in the delivery room to assist with the baby immediately after birth.

While it may be scary to think about using a specialist, these doctors have been specifically trained in caring for you and your baby. If it does become necessary to use a specialist for your care, try to remember that he or she has probably had a lot of experience working with other women in your same situation. You should always ask questions about processes and procedures you don't understand.

POTENTIAL RISKS

Gestational diabetes has the potential to cause significant complications that can affect your health and the health of your baby. It is important to work with your health care provider to carefully control your blood glucose levels to reduce the risk of certain complications. Nevertheless, there is a chance that you might be facing difficulties before, during, or after delivery of your baby.

Because diabetes can cause your baby to grow to be a large size, you may not carry your baby for the entire 40 weeks of pregnancy. As your baby grows larger, your doctor may watch you more carefully because the larger the size of the baby, the more difficult it can be to deliver. Having a baby that is very large can put you at risk of having tears in your vagina, cervix, or the skin of your perineum, which can be very painful. There is also the potential that these tears could bleed excessively, and sometimes a doctor may have to use stitches. After having a baby, your uterus normally contracts to slow the flow of blood. If you deliver a very large baby, your uterus could have problems contracting properly. In this case, you may need medication to cause your uterus to contract more, which can help to slow bleeding.

If you must deliver your baby early because he is getting too big, he is at risk of complications from prematurity. This can be confusing, because he may look like a normal-size baby who is the same as all of the other newborns in the nursery. However, he may act younger and have difficulties keeping his temperature regulated, feeding, or he may even have breathing difficulties if his lungs haven't fully matured. If this happens, your baby will need care from a doctor specializing in caring for premature newborns, typically a neonatologist, to ensure that he is kept warm, is eating well, and is not having any other health problems.

A large baby also can cause other problems during delivery. At times, a baby may have trouble being delivered and the doctor may need to use assistive devices such as forceps or a vacuum extractor to help. There are times when the baby can become injured while being born because of his size; one of the most common types of injuries is a broken collarbone when the baby has difficulty passing through the birth canal. Many women need to have a C-section in order to safely deliver their babies, but this is a surgical procedure that has the potential for risks in itself.

Your baby could also have difficulties maintaining a normal blood sugar level after he is born. He may need to be monitored closely by the nurses and have more frequent blood glucose checks to ensure that his blood sugar levels are within normal range. At times, some babies need assistance with feeding through a special feeding tube or an intravenous line to make sure that their blood sugar levels do not drop too low.

Delivering a baby can be difficult enough even when there are not any complications. It can be scary to think about having trouble, especially if everything is happening fast and a lot of people are taking care of you at the same time. Try to remain calm and remember that you are working with professionals who most likely have experience with these situations. If at all possible, monitor and control your blood glucose and take charge of your health during pregnancy to reduce the chance of complications.

MEDICAL INTERVENTION

Doctors and nurses have learned the steps to take to manage complications if they develop with your pregnancy or delivery. If you develop problems, follow the instructions from your doctor or midwife to work toward the best possible outcome.

Gestational diabetes puts you at risk of delivering your baby early. Uncontrolled high blood sugar levels may cause you to go into labor early, resulting in a preterm delivery. Alternatively, your doctor may induce labor early if your baby is growing too large for his age or is otherwise having difficulties. Preterm delivery puts your baby at risk of having respiratory distress. Because the lungs are one of the last organs to fully develop in the womb, a baby born before his due date is at risk of breathing problems because the lungs may be immature. If this happens, your baby may need help with breathing, such as with extra oxygen or tubing in the mouth or nose that delivers air to the lungs. He may need care in a specialized nursery where the nurses are trained in caring for premature babies. You can work with the doctors and nurses caring for your baby by following instructions to keep the environment safe and clean.

If your baby develops low blood sugar after birth, he may need help with eating to keep his blood glucose up. If you are breastfeeding, a nurse may have you try and help your baby to latch on right away. Alternatively, if your baby has significantly low blood sugar, he may need supplemental glucose through formula or an IV. A baby born to a mother with gestational diabetes may be more likely to have blood sugar problems after birth because he has been getting nutrients and glucose from his mother through the placenta. After delivery, his own body now has to create enough glucose to sustain his cells, but he may not be able to keep up right away. The nurses will check your baby's glucose and take steps to keep his blood sugar within the normal range. Although it may not be easy to watch your baby have lab tests or supplemental feedings, it is better than risking his blood sugar levels going too low.

Gestational diabetes is also associated with high blood pressure, which can put you at risk of pre-eclampsia. This condition occurs if your blood pressures are consistently high and you start to lose protein through your urine. The condition usually occurs after 20 weeks' gestation and could lead to problems with bleeding from the placenta, seizures, or lack of oxygen to the small vessels, including the brain. If a woman develops significant pre-eclampsia, she may need medication to control her blood pressure. In some cases, bed rest is also needed to avoid activities that can raise blood pressure or that could cause too much stimulation for the uterus.

Pre-eclampsia is a scary situation because in some cases, the only way to treat the condition is to deliver the baby early. This can put your baby at risk of complications of prematurity, such as breathing difficulties, an increased risk of jaundice, feeding problems, a greater risk of infection, and issues with controlling body temperature and gaining weight.

Notify your doctor if you develop any symptoms that may indicate that you have high blood pressure during your pregnancy. Some women have more swelling in the hands and feet, headaches, nausea and vomiting in the second or third trimester, sudden weight gain, or changes in vision. In many cases, pre-eclampsia has no symptoms at all and is only indicated by an increase in blood pressure levels. This is why it is important to attend all of your prenatal visits to have your blood pressure checked and to ensure that you continue to stay healthy.

THE EFFECTS OF TREATMENT ON OTHERS

Gestational diabetes may not only cause physical problems with your health and your baby's health, but it can also have an emotional impact on you and those involved in your pregnancy and care. Many women struggle with feelings of stress and depression after a diabetes diagnosis. It can be difficult to try and care for yourself while pregnant as well as check your blood sugar levels regularly and make changes to your diet and lifestyle. If you develop complications, it can feel overwhelming to go to appointments and have tests and procedures without knowing what is going on.

Your spouse or significant other may also have difficulty dealing with a gestational diabetes diagnosis. Family members may not understand the need for extra tests and procedures and it can be difficult to try and explain everything, especially if you are struggling to make sense of it yourself. You may need extra support for help with going to appointments, keeping schedules, or even providing child care if you have other children in the home. Some women have trouble trying to stay positive and upbeat when they do not feel well or when they are uncertain about some aspects of their pregnancy.

If you have difficulties with delivery or your baby needs specialized care after birth, you may feel saddened by missing those initial moments right after birth, especially if your baby was whisked away for care from a nurse or doctor. Many women worry about bonding with their infants after birth when further health care is needed, fearing that a bond is disrupted because of separation. However, most women are able to successfully bond with their infants when they are able to have time with them. Remember that bonding is a process, not a one-time event. Once your baby is stable, you will have many moments with him to care for and meet his needs as his mother.

Additionally, if you are feeling stressed or distant from family or your partner because of gestational diabetes, take time to talk things out with those who are important to you. Spend time together on activities that are unrelated to pregnancy and just try to have fun. Discuss your concerns and feelings and if necessary, seek outside help from a counselor or trusted friend who can help you sort through these sometimes-difficult emotions.

NUTRITIONAL MANAGEMENT

Good nutrition is so important for the management of gestational diabetes. Not only can following a healthy diet help you to control your blood glucose levels, it may also help with weight loss and you will be more likely to feel good because you are getting essential vitamins and nutrients from your food.

If you have been diagnosed with gestational diabetes, you may have a chance to talk with a dietician or diabetes educator about what type of diet to follow. A diabetic diet is one that follows a healthy eating plan of increased amounts of fruits, vegetables, and whole grains while limiting the amount of processed and refined carbohydrates and sugars. A diabetic eating plan is not necessarily a low-carbohydrate plan. Instead, the eating plan considers the carbohydrates that you do eat to make sure that you are taking in those that will give you energy as well as important nutrients.

Most foods consist of a blend of proteins, carbohydrates, and fats. Each of these substances are processed a little differently in the body. Protein is found in animal-based products such as meat and eggs, as well as some legumes, such as beans. A food that mostly contains protein may have little effect on your blood sugar, but many foods that have a lot of protein are often combined with other foods that contain carbohydrates or fats, such as certain sauces, gravies, or breading.

Protein is important for your health because it supports muscle tissue and keeps many of your hormones working properly. Protein is also an important component of healing of the body's tissues. Talk with your doctor or dietician about how much protein you should be eating daily, although most women who are pregnant and have GDM should take in between 6 and 8 oz. a day. Some examples of the best sources of protein include:

- Poultry (chicken or turkey)
- Lean beef
- Peanut butter
- Tofu
- Eggs
- Cheese
- Pork
- Seafood

THE GLYCEMIC INDEX AND GLYCEMIC LOAD

Certain foods raise your blood sugar after you eat; how much and how quickly your blood sugar rises after a meal depends on the glycemic index (GI) of a food. The GI is a type of ranking system that assigns a number to each food for how it affects blood sugar. Foods that have a high GI are digested quickly and cause your blood sugar to rise quickly. Alternatively, foods with a lower GI can help to keep your blood sugar levels more stable because they do not cause such a rapid rise. When choosing carbohydrate foods, try to pick those foods that have a low GI when compared with those with a high GI. Low GI foods are those with a score of less than 55. Some examples of foods that fall into this category are:

- Whole grain or pumpernickel bread
- Whole wheat pasta
- Beans and lentils
- Milk, yogurt, low-fat ice cream
- Apples, pears, strawberries, blueberries
- Corn, peas

Medium GI foods have scores between 56 and 69. You can sometimes add these foods to your diet. Examples are:

- Pita bread, taco shells
- Wild rice, couscous
- Sweet potatoes
- Cherries, pineapple, raisins
- Popcorn

High GI foods have scores between 70 and 100. You can eat these foods, but they should be added less often and in limited quantities. Some examples of high GI foods are:

- Instant oatmeal, sugared cereals
- White bread, English muffins, rice cakes
- Canned pasta, white rice
- Watermelon, canned fruit in heavy syrup
- Pretzels, cookies

Because portion sizes are also important, the glycemic load (GL) has been developed to better determine how quickly your glucose rises when you eat a serving of food. Calculating the glycemic load of food requires you to know how many carbohydrates are in each serving and multiply it by its glycemic index, then divide the number by 100. For example, if you eat a serving of crackers that has 20 g of carbohydrates and has a GI of 87, you can divide that by 100 to get 17.4. If your GL was less than 10, this is considered a low GL. A medium GL is 11 to 20, and more than 20 is high. Add all of your results up at the end of the day to determine how much glycemic load you should have each day. Your total number should not be more than 120.

Some people believe that because they have diabetes, they should not eat carbohydrates. Carbohydrates contribute to blood glucose levels when these types of foods are digested and processed in the gastrointestinal system. Depending on the type and amount of carbohydrates you eat, your blood sugar could rise quickly and stay elevated for quite some time after your meal. It is important to eat carbohydrates in order for your body's cells to get the energy they need. If possible, try to eat foods with carbohydrates throughout the day's meals and snacks. Your body may also respond well if you combine carbohydrates with protein when you eat, as this may have a less drastic effect on your blood sugar.

There are some carbohydrate-rich foods that you should avoid because they do not contribute nutrients to you or your baby and they have high levels of fat or sugar. Examples of some of these foods include cakes, candy, pastries, soft drinks, cookies, or potato chips. Eat these foods sparingly and only as a treat once in a while in small amounts.

When choosing what types of carbohydrate foods to eat, choose those that have a low glycemic index. Depending on your overall health and weight, you may need between 12 and 16 servings of carbohydrates per day. One serving is equal to 15 grams of carbohydrates. Examples of one serving of carbohydrates include:

- 1 slice of bread
- ½ English muffin
- ¾ cup cooked oatmeal
- ½ cup noodles
- 1 medium potato
- 1 medium apple, pear, or orange
- 1 ½ tablespoons of raisins
- 2 scoops of plain, low-fat ice cream

Most vegetables are very low in carbohydrates and will not have a strong impact on your blood glucose levels. When you prepare a meal, try to make half of your plate consist of non-starchy vegetables, which are low in calories and will provide many essential nutrients to you and your baby. Some types of vegetables that are tasty and very low in carbohydrates include:

- Asparagus
- Broccoli
- Cabbage
- Cucumber
- Eggplant
- Leeks
- Lettuce
- Pumpkin
- Radishes
- Spinach
- Tomatoes
- Zucchini

When preparing your vegetables, it is tempting to add creamy or buttery sauces to add flavor to the dish. While this tastes delicious, it can add calories and carbohydrates, and can add to the glycemic index of your food. There are many flavorful spices and seasonings that you can add, though, that contain less sugar, salt, and fat to your vegetables, such as chili, garlic, ginger, lemon, lime, or soy sauce.

Knowing what foods to eat and the effects of certain foods on your blood sugar can help you to better plan your meals. There are many options for healthy foods to incorporate into your diet, even if they are new or different than what you have experienced. Relax and have fun trying new foods; you may find a healthy treat that you truly enjoy.

The Next Steps

Testing for GDM is an essential part of the process for caring for your health during pregnancy. You may feel overwhelmed or as if you have little control over what happens, especially if you have been diagnosed with gestational diabetes. It is important to remember, though, that there are many things you can do to take charge of your health. Consider each of these steps and by incorporating them into your daily life, you are on your way toward a healthy pregnancy.

1. *Monitor and control your blood glucose levels.* If you have been diagnosed with GDM, this process is essential to managing your diabetes and your health. Follow the directions given by your doctor about how and when to check your blood sugar levels and know your goals for a healthy outcome. If you are having difficulties meeting your goals or you have any questions about the process of managing your blood sugar, talk with your health care provider.

2. *Follow a healthy diet and avoid gaining excess weight during your pregnancy.* With a better understanding of the importance of carbohydrates, protein, and fat in your diet as well as their effects on blood sugar, you can make many healthy choices of foods. If you are still unsure about the types of foods and amounts that you should eat, ask your health care provider for a referral to a dietician who can guide you and help you come up with a meal plan. You will have your weight checked regularly at your prenatal visits and your provider should give you guidelines about how much weight you can gain based on your pre-pregnancy weight and your state of health.

3. *Participate in regular physical activity.* Increase your activity levels and get moving with an exercise routine that

can help strengthen your body throughout your pregnancy. Avoid those activities that might not be safe, but otherwise strive for at least 150 minutes of moderate-intensity exercise each week. Talk to your doctor about your exercise plans and whether your routine is safe and beneficial during pregnancy.

4. *Take medications as prescribed by your doctor.* Your provider may prescribe medications to help keep your blood sugar within a normal range. Take all of your medications as ordered and notify your doctor if you are suffering from side effects that impact how much you are able to take the medicine.

5. *Take steps to prepare for delivery.* Understanding the basics of a safe and healthy delivery can better prepare you for this upcoming time. Regular exercise can strengthen your body to better prepare you for delivery as well. Learn what you can about the process of delivery and make a plan for when you go to the hospital. Understanding the potential complications associated with delivery when you have GDM is also important in case the process does not go as planned.

Although a diabetes diagnosis may be overwhelming during your pregnancy, there are many positive choices you can make to take care of yourself. Following through with testing, following your doctor's orders for treatment, and making the necessary lifestyle changes can all greatly increase your chances for a healthy pregnancy and a great outcome for both you and your baby.

OTHER BOOKS IN THE GESTATIONAL DIABETES SERIES:

Gestational Diabetes Diet Meal Plan and Recipes: Your Guide To Controlling Blood Sugars & Weight Gain (Baby Steps For Gestational Diabetes) (Volume 1)

http://www.amazon.com/Gestational-Diabetes-Diet-Meal-Recipes/dp/0615747736/

Gestational Diabetes Journal: Keeping Your Baby Healthy (Baby Steps For Gestational Diabetes) (Volume 2)

http://www.amazon.com/Gestational-Diabetes-Journal-Keeping-Healthy/dp/0615873928/

My Pregnancy Care with Gestational Diabetes: Tips on Diet, Grocery Shopping and Eating Out (Volume 4)

http://www.amazon.com/My-Pregnancy-Care-Gestational-Diabetes-ebook/dp/B00GPWYELI/

Life After Gestational Diabetes: 14 Ways To Reverse Your Risk Of Type 2 Diabetes (Baby Steps For Gestational Diabetes) (Volume 5)

http://www.amazon.com/Life-After-Gestational-Diabetes-Reverse-ebook/dp/B00FZEGRXA/

www.ingramcontent.com/pod-product-compliance
Lightning Source LLC
Chambersburg PA
CBHW060521280326
41933CB00014B/3062